THE GOLDEN YEARS: NUTRITION FOR WOMEN

The Ultimate Nutrition Guide for Women Over 40 with Secret Anti Aging Hacks

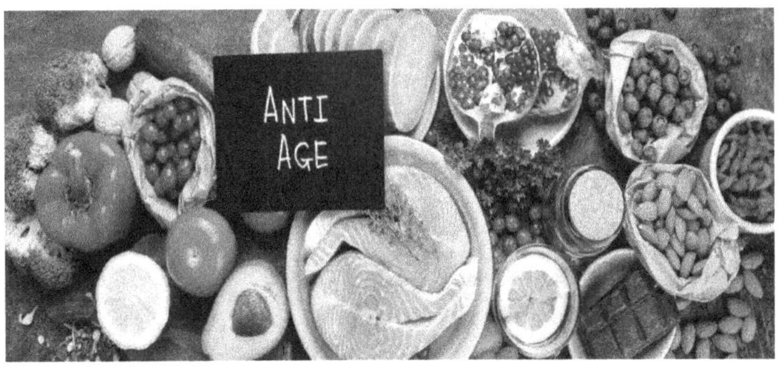

BENJAMIN AARON

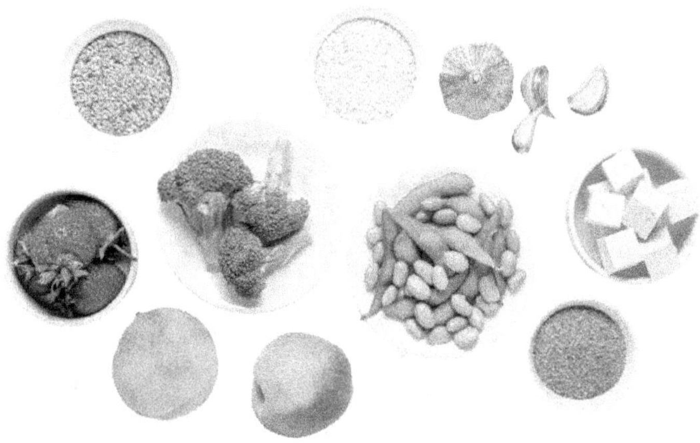

TABLE OF CONTENTS

INTRODUCTION

Mrs. Sophia was a 45 year old woman who had been struggling with the changes that come with menopause and aging. She had tried different diets and lifestyle changes but nothing seemed to help. Then, one day she stumbled upon a book called "The Golden Years: Nutrition for Women Over 40".

Mrs. Sophia decided to give it a try, and was amazed to find that the book contained practical advice that she could easily incorporate into her life. She learned how to make healthier food choices and develop a more balanced diet. She also learned how to make exercise an enjoyable part of her life.

Mrs. Sophia was delighted to find that the book gave her the knowledge and confidence to make positive changes in her life. She began to eat more nutrient-dense foods, cut back on processed foods, and started to incorporate more fresh fruits and vegetables into her meals. She also began to exercise regularly, taking long walks and doing simple yoga poses. After a few weeks of following the advice in the book, Mrs. Sophia began to feel better than ever before. She had more energy and felt stronger. The changes in her diet had made a huge difference in her overall health and wellbeing. Mrs. Sophia had successfully beaten menopause, aging and all its related changes. She was delighted to have found the book and was grateful for the knowledge and confidence it had given her. She now knew how to take care of herself and make healthy decisions for her body and mind. She was proud of herself for making such positive changes and was excited to see what the future held.

Welcome to Nutrition for Women Over 40! In this book, you will learn how to maintain optimal health and wellness as you age. We all know that our bodies change as we get older, and this book is designed to help you understand the necessary nutritional changes that come with aging and provide you with the tools you need to make healthy choices.

You will learn about menopause and its related changes, the importance of a balanced diet and how to incorporate healthy eating habits into your lifestyle. We will explore the changes that occur in your body as you age and how to make the most of them. We will also discuss the essential vitamins, minerals, and other nutrients needed to maintain your health and energy levels. You will also learn about the different conditions and diseases that may affect women over 40, such as heart disease, osteoporosis, and diabetes. We will discuss how to reduce the risk of these conditions and how to manage them once they have been diagnosed.

This book will provide you with the necessary knowledge and guidance to make informed decisions about your health and nutrition. We will look at the different types of foods and supplements that can help you stay healthy and fit as you age. With this book, you will gain the confidence you need to make healthy and informed choices!

So, let's get started!

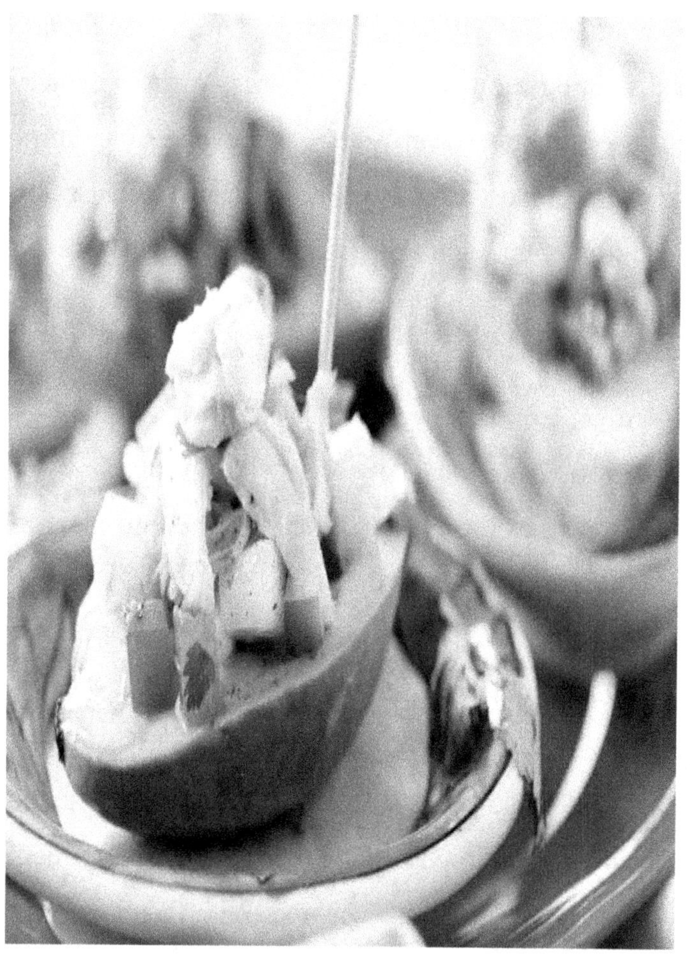

CHAPTER 1

MENOPAUSE AND ITS RELATED CHANGES

Menopause is the end of menstruation. The word menopause came from the Greek word "mens" meaning "monthly" and "pausis" meaning "cessation". Menopause is part of a woman's natural ageing process when her ovaries produce lover level of the estrogen and progesterone and when she is no longer able to become pregnant.

Menopause is a natural process in a woman's life when her body transitions from reproductive age to post-reproductive age. During this period, the body produces less of certain hormones, like estrogen and progesterone, and the body's reproductive system stops functioning. Menopause can cause a variety of physical, emotional, and psychological changes that can be disruptive to a woman's life. It is important for women to be aware of the changes that come with menopause and to seek help from healthcare professionals if needed.

PHASES OF MENOPAUSE

Menopause is broken down into four phases:-

1. **Pre-menopause:** The broad definition of premenopause is the time prior to menopause. The occurrence of menopause before the age of 40 years.

2. **Peri-menopause:** This is a period in women's life characterized by the physiological changes associated with the end of reproduction capacity and terminating with the completion of menopause. It is also called climacteric.

3. **Menopausal phase:** It is the end of menstrauation. The age of menopause ranges between 45 – 55 years, average being 50 years.

4. **Post – Menopausal Phase:** It is defined formally as the time after which a woman has experienced 12 consecutie months of amenorrhea without period.

INCIDENCE

Physiologic Menopause: The normal decline in ovarian function due to ageing begins in most women between ages 45 and 55, on average 51 and results in infrequent ovulation, decreased menstrual function and eventually cessation of menstruation.

Pathologic Menstruation: The gradual or abrupt cessation of menstruation before 40 years occurs idiopathically in about 5% of women in USA.

CAUSES OF MENOPAUSE

Menopause occurs when the ovaries are totally depleted of eggs, and no amount of stimulation from the regulating hormones can force them to work. This can result to the following changes in women:

1.   PHYSIOLOGICAL CHANGES

The lack of estrogen and progesterone causes many changes in women's physiology which also affect their health and well-being. The symptoms of menopause are due to the changes in the metabolism of the body.

- **Increased Cholesterol level in the blood:** Hyperlipidemia or an increase in the level of cholesterol and lipids in the blood is common. This leads to gradual rise in the risk of heart disease and stroke after menopause.

- **Osteoporosis:** The loss of calcium from the bone is increased in the first five years after the onset of menopause, resulting in a loss of bone density. The calcium moves out of the bones, leaving them weak and liable to fracture at the smallest stress.

- **Digestive System:** Motor activity of the entire digestive tract is diminished after menopause. The intestine tends to be sluggish, thereby resulting in constipation.

- **Urinary System:** As the estrogen level decreases after the menopause, the tissuenlining, the urethra and the bladder become drier, thinner and less elastic. This can lead to increases frequency of passing urine as well as an increased tendency of develop UTI (Urinary Tract Infection).

2.   CHANGES IN THE GENITAL ORGANS

- **The Uterus:** The uterus becomes small and fibrotic due to atrophy of the muscles after the menopause. The cervix becomes smaller and appears to flush with the vagina. In older women, the cervix may be impossible to identify separately from the vagina. The vagina and cervical discharge decreases in amount and later disappears completely.

- **Ovaries:** The ovaries become smaller and shriveled in appearance. The ovaries which produce little androgen during reproductive life begin to produce it in increasing amounts.

- **Vagina:** The vagina mucous membrane becomes thin and loses its rugosity after the menopause. Decreased secretion make vagina dry. Sexual intercourse becomes painful and difficult due to pain from the dry vagina.

- **Vulva or External Genital Organs:** The fat in the labia majora and the mons pubis decreases and pubic hair become sparse.

- **Breast:** In thin built women, the breast become flat and shriveled while in heavy built women, they become flabby and pendulous.

3. CHANGES IN GENERAL APPEARANCE

- **Skin:** The skin loses its elasticity and becomes thin and fine. This is due to the loss of elastin and collagen from the skin.
- **Weight:** Weight increase is more likely to be the result of irregular food habit due to mood swing. There is more desposition of fat around hips, waist and buttocks.
- **Hair:** Hair becomes dry and coarse after menopause. There may be hair loss due to the decreasing level of estrogen.
- **Voice:** Voice becomes deeper due to the thickening of vocal cords.

4. CHANGES IN THE VASOMOTOR SYSTEM

- **The Flashes:** Hot flashes are incidents where the women in menopause gets a sudden feeling of warmth and flushing that starts in the face and quickly spread all over the neck and upper body. They vary in number from 1 in every one hour to as one in every 15 minutes. The hot flashes are often associated with profuse sweating.

- **Night Sweat:** Night sweats are closely related to hot flashes. Both usually occurs simultabeously. Sweat can occur any time of the day or night but they are more common at night. The sweat can be severe enough to wake up the women from a sound sleep and may make it difficult for her to go back to sleep. The sudden waking up from sleep can cause palpitation and sometimes panic attacks.

5. PHYCHOLOGICAL CHANGES

The psychological changes are mainly

manifested by frequent headache, irritability, fatigue, depression and insomnia. Although, these are often said to be due to changes in the hormonal levels, they are more likely to be related to the loss of sleep due to night sweat. Diminished interest in sex may be due to emotional upset or may be secondary to painful intercourse due to a dry vagina.

6. SOCIAL CHANGES DURING MENOPAUSE

The feeling that a woman holds about herself and her social relationship as well as the syptoms she experiences can be defined by the culture in which she lives. Women vary in their subjective experiences of symptoms. Not all of the women's perceive changes in the body are reflected in the mirror; some are derived from women's perception of herself based on the account of other expectation vary and are adjusted to actual experience.

1. **NON – HORMONAL TREATMENT:**
   There are varieties of menopausal treatments both natural and medical that can alleviate the symptoms of menopause. Dressing in light layers can alleviate hot flashes and night sweats; avoid caffeine, alchohol and spicy foods can also minimize these symptoms. Menopause and weight gain tend to go together due to life syle changes than to the hormonal changes. Reducing dietary fat intake and regular exercise help to combat weight gain during menopause.

2. Menopause can lead to Osteoporosis. Calcium, magnesium and vitamin D can help restore bone density, which naturally deteriorates after age 30 due to reduced estrogen level. Menopause decreases vaginal elasticity, leading to vaginal dryness. Vitamin E can help as can regular exercises which help to restore elasticity. Using water based lubricants during sexual intercourse also minimizes discomfort related to vaginal dryness.

3. Menopause often leads to dry, itchy skin, and weak thin hair that breaks and that has lots of split ends. Flax seed oil (fouud in poulty, diary, red meat and whole grains) can help restore hair and skin healthy appearance, as can vitamin E.

HORMONE REPLACEMENT THERAPY

Hormone replacement therapy (HRT) is indicated in menopausal women to overcome the short term and long term consequences of estrogen defiency. HRT can be admistered orally (in pill form), vaginally (as a cream), or transdermally (in patch form) because it replaces female hormones produced by the ovaries, hormone replacement therapy minimizes menopause sysptoms. It can be used before, during and after menopause. There are several indications of HRT which includes:

- Relief of menopausal symptoms
- Prevention of osteoporosis
- To maintain the quality of life in menopausal years

Special group of womento whom HRT should be prescribed include:

- Women with premature ovarian failure.
- Gonadal dysgenesis
- Surgical or radiation menopause.

Conclusively, menopause is a natural transition in a woman's life, marking the end of her reproductive years. It is the time when the ovaries stop releasing eggs and her menstrual cycle ceases. During this transition, women often experience a range of physical and psychological symptoms, including hot flashes, night sweats, vaginal dryness, and mood swings. While menopause is natural and unavoidable, there are some treatments available to help women manage the symptoms.

Hormone replacement therapy (HRT) is the most common form of treatment for menopausal symptoms. It replaces the diminishing hormones in a woman's body with synthetic ones. This can help reduce hot flashes and night sweats, as well as improves vaginal health. It can also help reduce the risk of osteoporosis and other complications related to menopause. However, HRT may come with some risks, including an increased risk of stroke and breast cancer, so it is important to discuss the risks and benefits with your doctor before starting any form of HRT.

Over-the-counter medications can also be used to help relieve menopausal symptoms. Non-hormonal medications, such as ibuprofen and acetaminophen, are often used to help reduce hot flashes and night sweats. Some herbal supplements, such as black cohosh and soy, may also help reduce menopausal symptoms. However, the effectiveness of these treatments is not well established, and it is best to discuss their use with your doctor before starting any of them.

Lifestyle changes can also be beneficial for managing menopausal symptoms. Eating a balanced diet and exercising regularly can help reduce hot flashes and other symptoms. Avoiding alcohol, caffeine, and spicy foods can also help reduce symptoms. Additionally, getting enough sleep and managing stress can help keep symptoms in check.

Finally, there are some alternative treatments available for menopausal symptoms. These include acupuncture, massage therapy, and hypnosis. These treatments have not been thoroughly studied, so it is important to discuss them with your doctor before trying any of them.

In conclusion, menopause is a natural transition in a woman's life, and it is important to discuss the various treatments available with your doctor before starting any of them. Hormone replacement therapy is the most common form of treatment for menopausal symptoms, but there are also over-the-counter medications and lifestyle changes that can help. Additionally, there are some alternative treatments available, such as acupuncture and massage therapy, but their effectiveness has not been thoroughly studied. It is important to discuss all of your options with your doctor before starting any treatment.

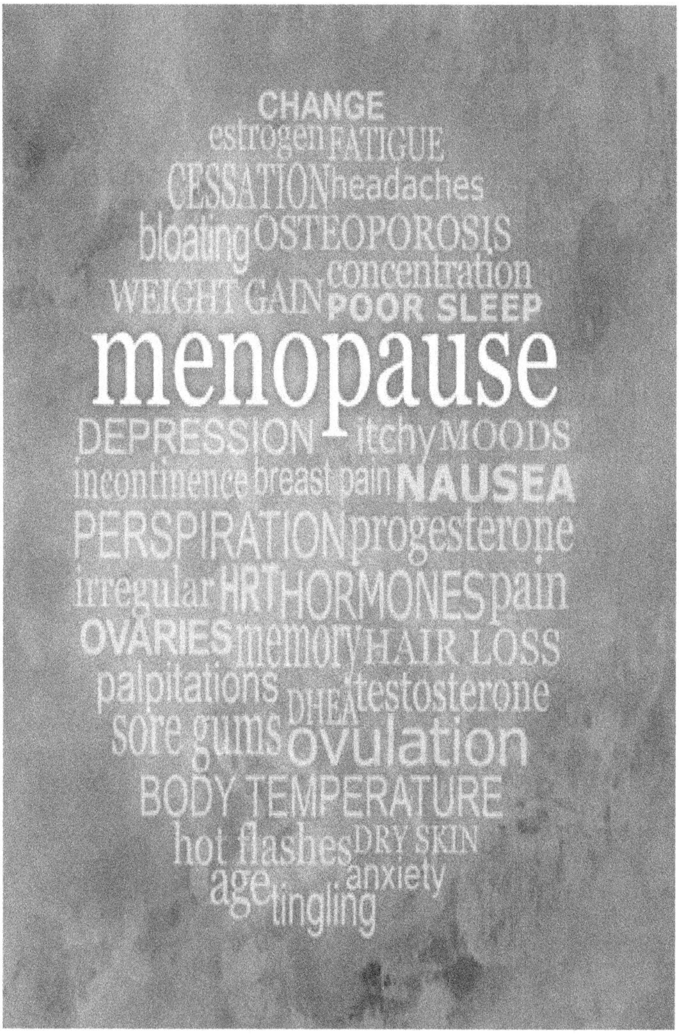

CHANGE
estrogen FATIGUE
CESSATION headaches
bloating OSTEOPOROSIS
concentration
WEIGHT GAIN POOR SLEEP
menopause
DEPRESSION itchy MOODS
incontinence breast pain NAUSEA
PERSPIRATION progesterone
irregular HRT HORMONES pain
OVARIES memory HAIR LOSS
palpitations DHEA testosterone
sore gums ovulation
BODY TEMPERATURE
hot flashes DRY SKIN
age anxiety
tingling

CHAPTER 2

NUTRITIONAL NEEDS OF WOMEN OVER 40

Women over 40 have different nutritional needs than younger women, due to changes in metabolism, hormones, and lifestyle. As women age, their nutrient needs become more complex and it is important to ensure they receive the right combination of nutrients to maintain good health and prevent chronic disease. Eating a well-balanced diet with a variety of nutrient-rich foods is essential for women over 40 to meet their unique nutritional needs. This includes plenty of fruits and vegetables, lean proteins, whole grains, low-fat dairy and healthy fats. Supplements may also be beneficial for some women, depending on their dietary habits and nutritional needs. In addition to eating a healthy diet, women over 40 should engage in regular physical activity to maintain muscle and bone strength, prevent weight gain, and reduce the risk of chronic diseases. By understanding the unique nutritional needs of women over 40 and how to meet them, you can ensure that you are getting the nutrients you need for optimal health and wellness. The following are some of the key nutritional needs of women over 40:

1. **Protein:** Women over 40 need to increase their protein intake to maintain muscle mass, which tends to decline with age. The recommended daily allowance (RDA) for protein is 46 grams for women over 40. Adequate protein is essential for the growth, repair, and maintenance of muscle and other tissues. Women over 40 should focus on consuming high-quality proteins such as fish, poultry, legumes, eggs, nuts, and seeds.

2. **Calcium:** Women over 40 are at greater risk for osteoporosis, so it is important to ensure adequate calcium intake. The RDA for calcium is 1,000 mg per day for women over 40, and can be obtained from low-fat dairy products like yogurt, cheese, and milk, as well as from green leafy vegetables, nuts, and fish.

3. **Iron:** Women over 40 are at greater risk for iron deficiency anemia due to menstrual blood loss, so it is important to ensure adequate iron intake. The RDA for iron is 8 mg per day for women over 40 and can be obtained from lean meats, poultry, fish, and fortified grains and cereals.

4. **Vitamin D:** Vitamin D is important for bone health and helps the body absorb calcium. The RDA for Vitamin D is 600 IU per day for women over 40 and can be obtained from fortified dairy products, fatty fish, and eggs.

5. **Fiber:** Fiber helps to keep the digestive system healthy and promote regularity. The RDA for fiber is 25-30 grams per day for women over 40 and can be obtained from whole grains, fruits, vegetables, legumes, and nuts.

6. **Omega-3 Fatty Acids:** Omega-3 fatty acids are important for heart health and can be obtained from fatty fish like salmon, sardines, and tuna. The recommended

daily allowance for omega-3 fatty acids is 1.1-1.6 grams per day for women over 40.

7. **Folic Acid:** Folic acid is important for cellular health and can be obtained from fortified grains, legumes, leafy green vegetables, and citrus fruits. The recommended daily allowance for folic acid is 400 mcg per day for women over 40.

8. **Magnesium:** Magnesium is important for nerve and muscle health and can be obtained from nuts, legumes, and whole grains. The recommended daily allowance for magnesium is 320 mg per day for women over 40.

9. **Vitamin B12:** Vitamin B12 is important for cognitive and neurological health and can be obtained from fortified grains, foods containing animal proteins, and dietary supplements. The recommended daily allowance for Vitamin B12 is 2.4 mcg per day for women over 40.

10. **Vitamin A:** Vitamin A is important for vision and can be obtained from orange and yellow fruits and

vegetables, as well as from fortified dairy products. The recommended daily allowance for Vitamin A is 700 mcg per day for women over 40.

11. **Water:** Adequate hydration is essential for overall health and well-being. Women over 40 should aim to drink at least 8 cups of water per day.

12. **Limit Alcohol Intake:** Alcohol can have a detrimental effect on overall health, so it is important to limit intake. The recommended daily limit for alcohol is one drink per day for women over 40.

13. **Limit Caffeine Intake:** Caffeine can have a detrimental effect on overall health, so it is important to limit intake. The recommended daily limit for caffeine is 400 mg per day for women over 40.

14. **Regular Exercise:** Regular exercise helps to maintain muscle mass and strength, promote heart health, and reduce the risk of some chronic diseases. Women over 40 should aim to get at least 30 minutes of

moderate exercise most days of the week.

15. **Stress Management:** Stress can have a detrimental effect on overall health, so it is important to practice stress management techniques like yoga, meditation, and deep breathing. Also, make sure to get enough sleep and engage in activities that bring joy and relaxation.

16. **Healthy Eating Habits:** Eating a balanced diet that is rich in whole foods like fruits, vegetables, lean proteins, and whole grains can help to ensure that women over 40 are getting all the essential nutrients they need. Also, limiting processed and refined foods and avoiding excessive amounts of sugar and saturated fat can help to promote overall health.

17. **Supplementation:** If needed, women over 40 can supplement their diet with a multivitamin and mineral supplement to ensure they are getting all the essential nutrients they need. However, it is important to speak to a healthcare professional before beginning any supplementation program.

The nutritional needs of women over 40 are complex and require a balanced, nutrient-rich diet to ensure their health and well-being. As women age, their body composition and metabolism change, and they require more nutrients and fewer calories. They need adequate amounts of carbohydrates, protein, fat, vitamins, minerals, and water to maintain good health.

Calcium is particularly important for women over 40, as they are at higher risk of developing osteoporosis. Eating foods rich in calcium, such as dairy products, green leafy vegetables, and some fish, is essential. Adequate fiber is also important, as fiber helps regulate digestion and can help lower the risk of certain diseases. Eating a variety of fruits and vegetables can provide fiber, as well as essential vitamins and minerals.

Women over 40 should also pay attention to their intake of saturated fat and added sugar. Eating too much-saturated fat can increase the risk of heart disease, while foods high in added sugar can cause weight gain and blood sugar issues.

In conclusion, women over 40 need a balanced diet to ensure their health and well-being. This diet should include adequate amounts of carbohydrates, protein, fat, vitamins, minerals, and water, as well as fiber and calcium. Eating a variety of fruits and vegetables, limiting saturated fat and added sugar intake, and staying hydrated can help ensure that women over 40 get the nutrients they need.

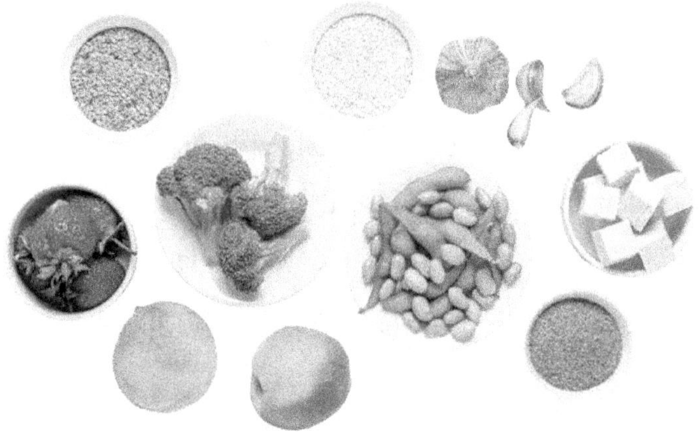

CHAPTER 3

HEALTHY EATING STRATEGIES

A woman's diet is one of the most important factors in her overall health and wellness. Women over 40 need to pay special attention to their diets in order to stay healthy and maintain a healthy weight. Eating healthy is not only important for physical health, but also for mental health. Eating well gives women the energy they need to stay active and productive throughout their day. Unfortunately, with age, come some nutritional challenges, such as food intolerances, digestive problems, and changes in metabolism. Eating a balanced diet is essential at any age, but for women over 40, it is especially important to choose nutrient-dense foods that provide the most nourishment. To ensure that women over 40 are getting the nutrition they need, they should follow certain healthy eating strategies.

Here are some healthy eating strategies for women over 40:

EAT A VARIETY OF WHOLE FOODS

Eating a variety of whole, unprocessed foods is essential for a healthy diet. This means avoiding processed and refined foods, such as white bread and white sugar, and instead opting for whole grain bread and natural sweeteners, like honey and maple. syrup. Focus on consuming a wide variety of fruits and vegetables, legumes, nuts and seeds, lean proteins, and healthy fats. This will ensure that you are getting the most nutrient-dense foods possible.

LIMIT SUGAR AND REFINED CARBS

Too much sugar and refined carbohydrates can lead to weight gain, fatigue, and blood sugar imbalances. Try to limit your intake of processed and refined foods, such as white bread, white rice, and sugary snacks and drinks. Instead, opt for whole grain bread and pasta and natural sweeteners, like honey or maple syrup.

INCREASE YOUR INTAKE OF HEALTHY FATS

Healthy fats, such as those found in avocados, nuts, and fatty fish, are essential for a healthy diet. These fats not only provide energy and help you feel fuller for longer, but they are also important for hormone production and maintaining healthy skin and hair.

ADD MORE FIBER TO YOUR DIET

Increasing your fiber intake is essential for digestive health, as well as for maintaining a healthy weight. Eating plenty of fruits, vegetables, and whole grains is an easy way to increase your fiber intake. Alternatively, you can opt for fiber supplements, such as psyllium husk or chia seeds.

STAY HYDRATED

Staying hydrated is the key for overall health and wellness. Make sure to drink plenty of water throughout the day and limit your intake of sugary drinks and caffeinated beverages.

GET ENOUGH SLEEP

Getting enough sleep is essential for good health. Aim for seven to eight hours of sleep per night, and try to go to bed and wake up at the same time each day.

EXERCISE REGULARLY

Exercise is important for maintaining a healthy weight and for overall health and well-being. Aim for at least 30 minutes of physical activity most days of the week.

In addition to eating a balanced diet, women over 40 should also pay attention to portion sizes. Any food consumed in excess might result in weight gain and other health issues. To keep portion sizes in check, women should be mindful of their hunger levels and only eat until they feel full. They should also try to measure their food portions using a food scale or measuring cups. This will help them to ensure that they are eating the right amount of food.

They may also benefit from incorporating certain superfoods into their diet. Superfoods are foods that are particularly nutrient-dense and provide a variety of health benefits. Some examples of superfoods include fish, legumes, nuts, seeds, and dark leafy greens. Incorporating these foods into meals can help to boost overall nutrition levels and provide the body with the necessary vitamins and minerals it needs.

By following these healthy eating strategies, women over 40 can ensure that they are getting the nutrients they need to stay healthy and maintain a healthy weight. Eating a variety of nutrient-dense whole foods, limiting sugar and refined carbohydrates, increasing your intake of healthy fats, adding more fiber to your diet, staying hydrated, getting enough sleep, and exercising regularly are all essential for a healthy diet.

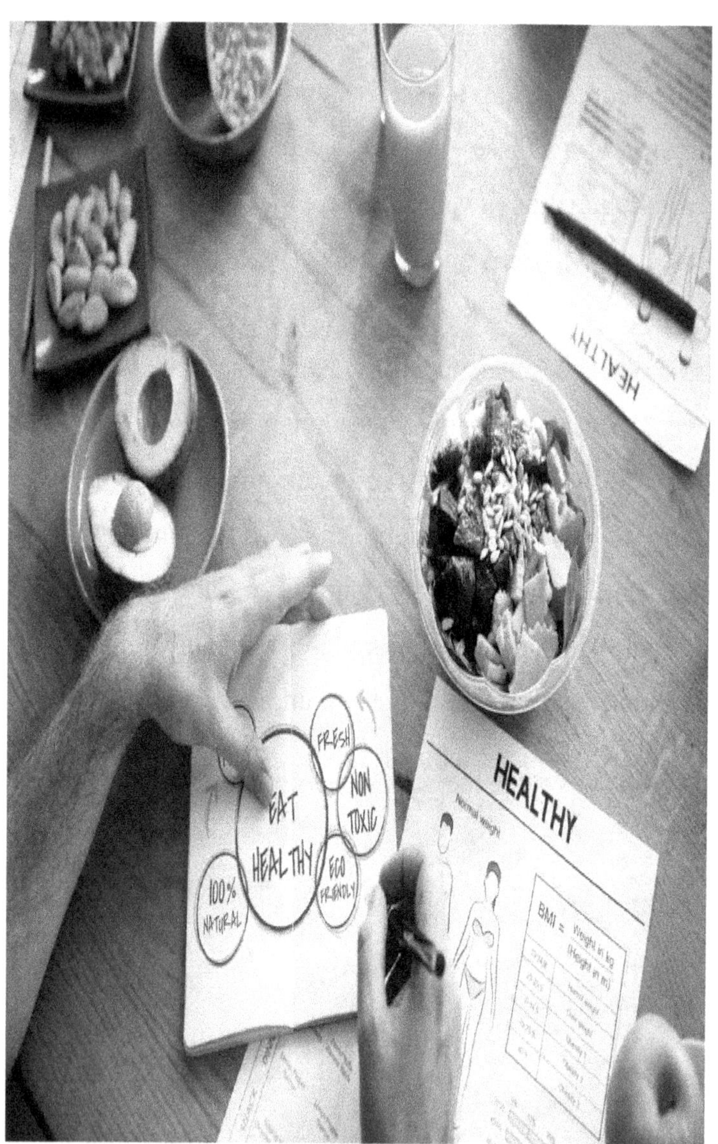
FRESH
NON TOXIC
EAT
HEALTHY
100%
NATURAL
ECO FRIENDLY
HEALTHY
Normal weight
BMI = Weight in kg
(Height in m)²

CHAPTER 4

MEAL PLANNING

Meal planning can be an important part of any woman's life, but it is especially important for women over 40. Planning your meals in advance can help you maintain a healthy weight and provide you with the energy and nutrients you need to stay healthy. Meal planning can also help you save time and money by reducing the amount of time you spend shopping for food and eating out.

For women over 40, it's important to focus on nutrient-dense foods that provide the most nutritional bang for your buck. This means focusing on whole grains, fruits, vegetables, lean proteins, healthy fats, and dairy products. You should also aim to include foods from all five food groups in each meal. Eating a balanced diet can help you stay energized throughout the day and reduce your risk of chronic diseases such as diabetes, heart disease, and certain cancers.

When planning your meals, it's important to think about the types of foods you'll be eating and the portion sizes you'll need. Eating smaller meals more frequently throughout the day can help you maintain an even energy level and keep you feeling fuller for longer. When choosing your meals, it's important to try to focus on fresh, minimally processed foods. This means buying locally grown produce, buying organic whenever possible, and avoiding processed meats, canned soups, and boxed meals. It's also important to make sure that you're including a variety of different foods in each meal to ensure that you're getting the full range of essential vitamins and minerals.

When it comes to meal planning, it's important to plan ahead and be flexible. Plan out your meals for the week and make sure you have enough food in your pantry and refrigerator to last you until your next grocery trip. Try to make a larger batch of a meal so that you can use it for multiple meals during the week. It's also a good idea to make a grocery list before you go to the store to make sure you're only buying what you need.

Meal planning can also help you save money by reducing the amount of food you throw away. It's important to use up leftovers within a few days and freeze any extra food you don't plan to eat right away. You should also plan to make meals that use up food you already have in your pantry and refrigerator, such as a stir-fry or soup.

In addition to planning your meals, it's also important to make sure you're getting enough physical activity. Aim to get at least 30 minutes of moderate exercise 5 days a week. Exercises such as jogging, walking, swimming, or biking are very essential. Exercise can help you maintain a healthy weight, reduce your risk of chronic diseases, and give you more energy throughout the day.

Below is a one-day balanced meal plan that women over 40 can try out.

BREAKFAST

- Oatmeal with banana slices and walnuts
- Scrambled eggs with spinach and mushrooms
- 1 cup of orange juice

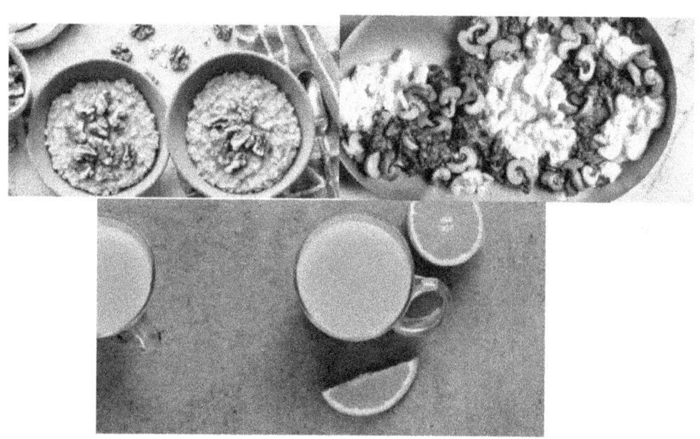

LUNCH

- Salad with grilled chicken, spinach, carrots, tomatoes, and feta cheese
- Baked sweet potato
- 1 cup of herbal tea

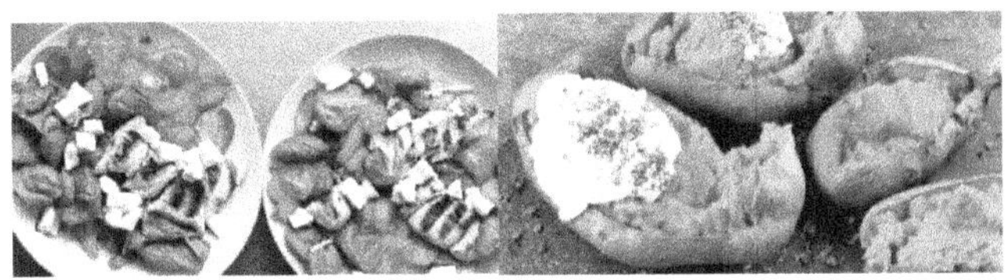

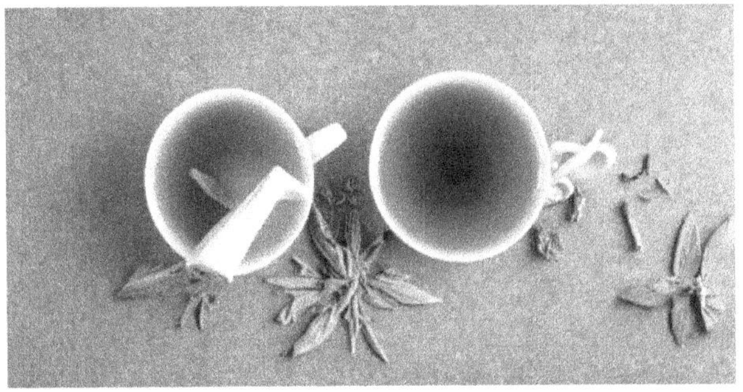

SNACK

Greek yogurt with berries and almonds

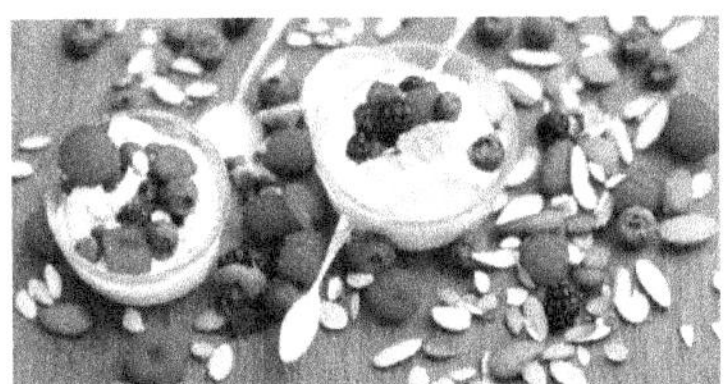

DINNER

- Grilled salmon with roasted vegetables and quinoa

- 1 glass of red wine

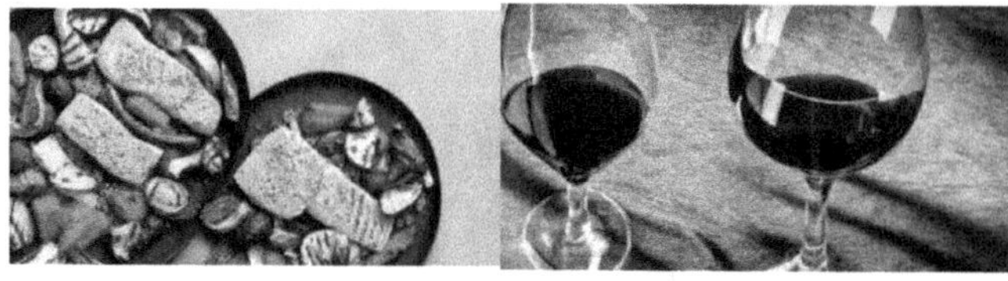

DESSERT

Fruit salad with a scoop of Greek yogurt

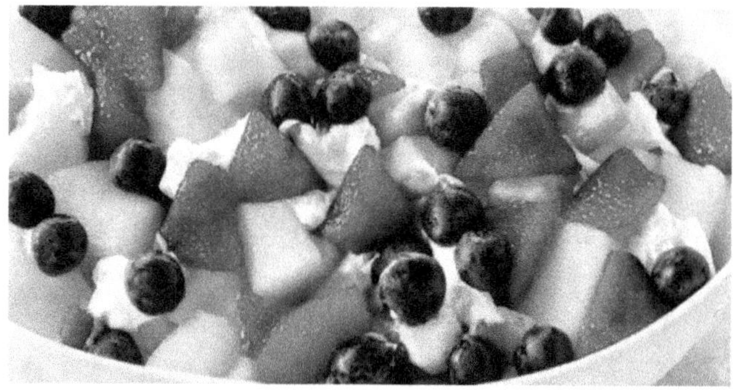

Discover more of my over 50 secret anti-aging recipe coupled with a 7-day meal plan hacks that will keep your health fresh and blooming. You can get these amazing recipes couple with their preparation instructions by searching for the copy of my book titled WEIGHT LOSS AFTER 60

CHAPTER 5

SUPERFOODS FOR OPTIMAL HEALTH

Superfoods for optimal health are nutrient-dense foods that provide a variety of essential vitamins, minerals, and other health-promoting nutrients. Examples of superfoods include blueberries, salmon, spinach, avocados, quinoa, chia seeds, and nuts. These foods are packed with antioxidants, omega-3 fatty acids, fiber, and other nutrients that can benefit overall health. Eating a variety of superfoods may help reduce the risk of chronic diseases such as heart disease, diabetes, and certain types of cancer.

In addition to a balanced diet, adding superfoods to your meals may help you to maintain a healthy weight and get the nutrients your body needs. Incorporating superfoods into your diet is an easy way to make sure you're getting enough of the essential nutrients that your body needs to stay healthy. Women over 40 have unique health needs that can be addressed through proper nutrition. Eating the right foods can help to improve overall health and well-being. Superfoods are nutrient-rich foods that are considered to be particularly beneficial for health and vitality. There are many superfoods that can help women over 40 maintain their health and vitality.

First, blueberries are considered a superfood due to their high concentration of antioxidants. Antioxidants help to fight off free radicals, which can cause damage to cells and contribute to the development of chronic diseases. Blueberries can be enjoyed as a snack or added to smoothies, cereal, and yogurt.

Second, salmon is an excellent source of omega-3 fatty acids, which are known to reduce inflammation and support heart health. Nuts and seeds such as walnuts, almonds, and chia seeds are other good sources of omega-3 fatty acids.

Third, dark leafy greens such as spinach, kale, and chard are packed with vitamins and minerals. They are also high in fiber, which can help to support digestion and reduce the risk of chronic diseases.

Fourth, legumes such as beans and lentils are a great source of protein, fiber, and other nutrients. They can be enjoyed as a side dish or added to soups and salads.

Fifth, avocados are a great source of healthy fats, which can help to lower cholesterol levels and reduce the risk of heart disease. They can be enjoyed as a snack or added to salads or sandwiches.

Sixth, whole grains such as oats, quinoa, and brown rice are good sources of fiber and essential vitamins and minerals. They can be enjoyed as a side dish or added to soups, salads, and casseroles.

Finally, Greek yogurt is a great source of protein and

probiotics, which can help to support digestion and reduce inflammation. It can be enjoyed as a snack or added to smoothies, oatmeal, and salads.

In conclusion, eating a diet rich in superfoods is an important part of maintaining optimal health for women over 40. Eating a variety of nutrient-rich foods can help to reduce the risk of chronic diseases and improve overall health and well-being.

CHAPTER 6

EATING OUT AND ON THE GO

Eating out and on the go is a term that refers to having meals away from home, usually in a restaurant, cafe, food truck, or other eating establishment. It can also mean having food delivered to your home or office or packing a meal to take to your destination. Because of the convenience and variety of options available, eating out and on the go has become increasingly popular in recent years. Eating out and on the go can be a great way to socialize with friends, family, and colleagues, or to enjoy a special occasion. It can also help to save time and money, as many restaurants offer discounts for eating out and on the go. Eating out and on the go can also be a healthier choice than eating at home due to the variety of quality and nutritious options available.

The primary advantage of eating out and on the go is convenience. Whether you are looking for a quick bite to eat for lunch, dinner, or a snack, eating out and on the go can provide you with a variety of options that are convenient and often reasonably priced. Eating out and on the go also allows you to enjoy the atmosphere of the restaurant or cafe, which can be a great way to relax and socialize. Additionally, many restaurants offer delivery services, making it even easier to enjoy a meal without the hassle of having to leave the comfort of your home.

When eating out and on the go, it is important to remember to make healthy choices and to be mindful of portion sizes and calories. It is also important to be aware of the potential risks associated with eating out, such as food contamination and cross-contamination. In addition, it is important to remember to practice safe food handling and preparation practices, such as washing hands and surfaces thoroughly and avoiding cross-contamination.

Women over 40 who eat out and/or eat on the go are

likely to experience common health concerns. Eating out and on the go can lead to an increased intake of unhealthy fats, added sugars, and sodium, as well as a decrease in essential vitamins and minerals. Additionally, an increase in portion sizes can lead to weight gain, which can increase the risk of developing chronic illnesses such as type-2 diabetes and heart disease. It can also lead to an increase in stress levels due to the lack of control over meal planning, which can further compound the health concerns associated with dietary changes. The following are other common health concerns facing women over 40:

1. Osteoporosis: Women over 40 are at higher risk for osteoporosis due to lower levels of estrogen and decreased bone density. This can be addressed through a balanced diet that includes plenty of calcium and vitamin D, weight-bearing exercise, and avoiding smoking and excessive alcohol consumption.

2. Heart Disease: Heart disease is a major concern for women over 40, and can be addressed through a healthy diet that is low in saturated fat and cholesterol, as well as regular exercise.

3. High blood pressure: High blood pressure is a common health concern for women over 40. It can be addressed through healthy eating habits such as decreasing salt intake, avoiding processed foods and saturated fats, and increasing fiber and whole grains.

4. Weight Gain: As women age, their metabolism slows, which can lead to weight gain. A healthy diet high in fiber and low in sugar, along with regular exercise, can help to prevent or reverse weight gain.

5. Diabetes: Women over 40 are at higher risk for diabetes. Eating a healthy, balanced diet and getting regular exercise can help to prevent and manage diabetes.

6. Breast Cancer: Women over 40 should talk to their doctor about getting regular mammograms, as well as performing self-exams to check for any suspicious lumps or changes in their breasts. Eating a healthy diet and avoiding excessive alcohol consumption can also help reduce the risk of breast cancer.

7. Menopause: Menopause can bring a variety of health concerns, including hot flashes, night sweats, mood swings, and decreased bone density. Eating a healthy diet that includes plenty of calcium and vitamin D, as well as regular exercise, can help reduce the symptoms of menopause.

8. Stress: Stress can affect women of all ages, but can be particularly detrimental for those over 40. Eating a healthy, balanced diet and getting regular physical activity can help reduce stress levels. Additionally, incorporating stress-reducing activities such as yoga or meditation can be beneficial.

9. Skin Changes: Skin changes can occur as a result of aging and can include wrinkles, age spots, and dryness. Eating a diet high in antioxidants can help protect the skin from damage. Additionally, using a good sunscreen and moisturizer can help reduce the signs of aging.

10. Cognitive Decline: Cognitive decline can be a concern for women over 40, and can be addressed through lifestyle changes such as eating a healthy diet, exercising regularly, and getting plenty of rest. Additionally, staying socially active and engaging in activities that challenge the brain can help to preserve cognitive function.

However, when informed nutritional decisions are given foremost priority, eating out and on the go can be especially beneficial, as it can provide a convenient way to have a nutritious meal. Many restaurants offer healthy options such as salads, grilled proteins, and whole grains. Additionally, many restaurants provide nutritional information on their menus, making it easier to make informed choices. The following are nutritional guidelines for women over 40 to help them make an informed choice when eating out and on the go:

1. Choose meals that are nutrient-dense, such as salads, grilled proteins, and whole grains.
2. Avoid fried and processed foods, as well as high-

calorie sauces and dressings.

3. Look for healthy preparation techniques, such as baking, grilling, and steaming.

4. Ask for dressings and sauces on the side to control portion size.

5. Ask for nutrition information when available.

6. Share an entrée or order a smaller portion size.

7. Choose whole fruits for dessert rather than pastries or other sugary treats.

8. Drink plenty of water and limit alcoholic beverages.

Following these guidelines can help ensure that you are making informed and healthy choices when eating out and on the go.

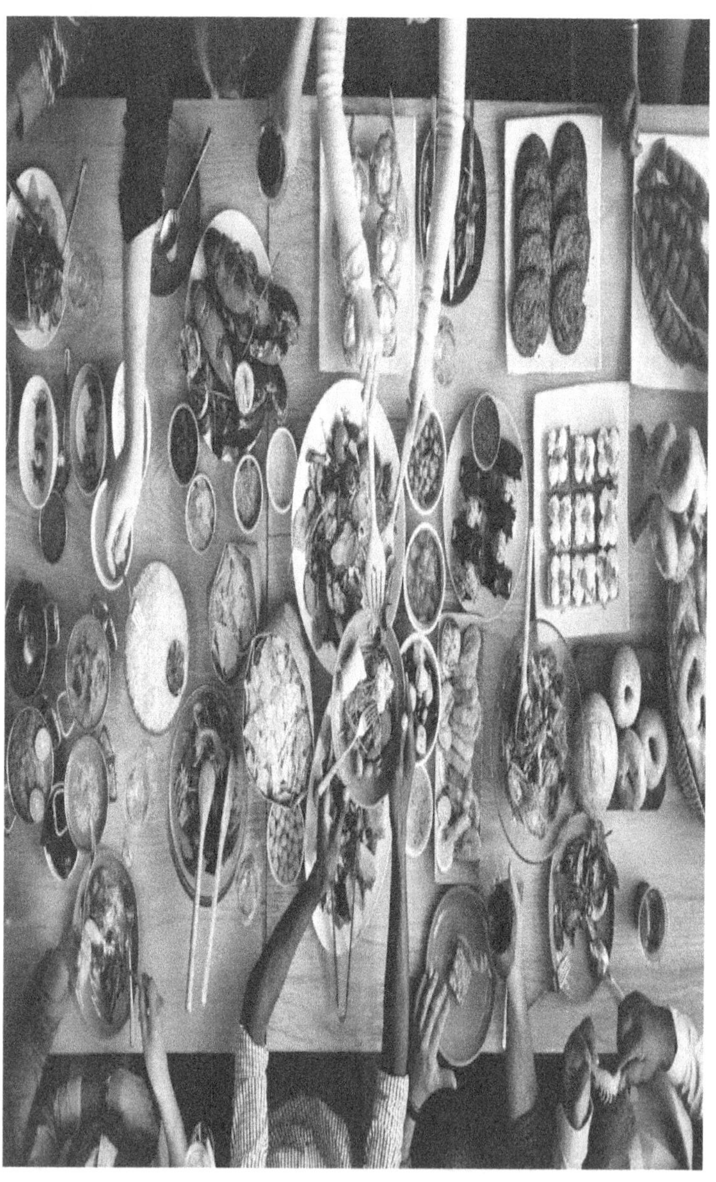

CHAPTER 7

SUPPLEMENTS AND HEALTHY AGING

Supplements are products that are taken to supplement or add to, the vitamins, minerals, and other nutrients found in the foods we eat. They are available as pills, capsules, powders, and liquids, among other forms. Supplements are not meant to replace a healthy diet, but rather to provide extra nutrients that may be lacking in our diets. They are often taken to address specific health concerns, such as deficiencies, or to enhance physical performance. Examples of supplements include multivitamins, omega-3 fatty acids, probiotics, and herbal remedies.

As people age, it is important to take steps to ensure that they maintain their health and well-being. One of the ways in which people can do this is by incorporating supplements into their diet. Supplements are substances that are meant to be taken orally in order to supplement the diet. They can come in the form of pills, capsules, powders, liquids, or even bars. When it comes to healthy aging, there are many different types of supplements that can be beneficial. For instance, people may want to consider taking vitamins and minerals such as vitamin C, vitamin D, zinc, and magnesium. These vitamins and minerals can help support the body's immune system, helping to ward off disease and infection. They can also help to support healthy bones, helping to prevent bone loss and fractures.

Additionally, people may want to consider taking supplements that contain omega-3 fatty acids. Omega-3 fatty acids can help support healthy brain function, which is especially important as people age. They can also help to reduce inflammation in the body, which can help to reduce the risk of chronic diseases such as arthritis and heart disease. Finally, people may want to consider taking supplements that contain antioxidants. Antioxidants can help to reduce the damage caused by free radicals, which can help to slow the aging process. They can also help reduce inflammation, and support healthy skin, hair, and nails.

In summary, taking supplements can be a great way to support healthy aging. By taking a variety of vitamins and minerals, omega-3 fatty acids, and antioxidants, people can help ensure that their bodies remain healthy and strong as they age.

The following are supplements that will necessitate a healthy aging for women over 40; viz:

1. **Multivitamin:** A multivitamin is a supplement that contains essential vitamins and minerals that help support optimal health.

2. **Omega-3 fatty acids:** Omega-3 fatty acids are essential for heart health, joint health, and brain health.

3. **Calcium:** Calcium is essential for bone health and helps to protect against bone loss associated with aging.

4. **Vitamin D:** Vitamin D helps to regulate calcium absorption and is important for healthy bones.

5. **B Vitamins:** B vitamins are important for energy

production and help combat fatigue.

6. **Probiotics:** Probiotics can help maintain digestive health and support the immune system.

7. **CoQ10:** CoQ10 is an antioxidant that helps protect cells from damage and may help reduce the risk of certain diseases.

8. **Antioxidants:** Antioxidants help to protect cells from damage caused by free radicals.

9. **Ginseng**: Ginseng is a popular herb that may help to reduce fatigue, improve mood, and reduce the effects of stress.

10. **Green tea extract:** Green tea extract is rich in antioxidants and may help reduce inflammation and boost the immune system.

11. **Resveratrol:** Resveratrol is an antioxidant that has been shown to help reduce the risk of certain diseases.

12. **Magnesium:** Magnesium is an essential mineral that helps to regulate blood pressure, support muscle and nerve function, and promote healthy sleep.

13. **Iron:** Iron is an essential mineral that helps to maintain healthy red blood cells and is important for energy production.

14. **Zinc:** Zinc is an essential mineral that helps to support the immune system and skin health.

15. **Selenium:** Selenium is an antioxidant that helps protect cells from damage and may help reduce the risk of certain diseases.

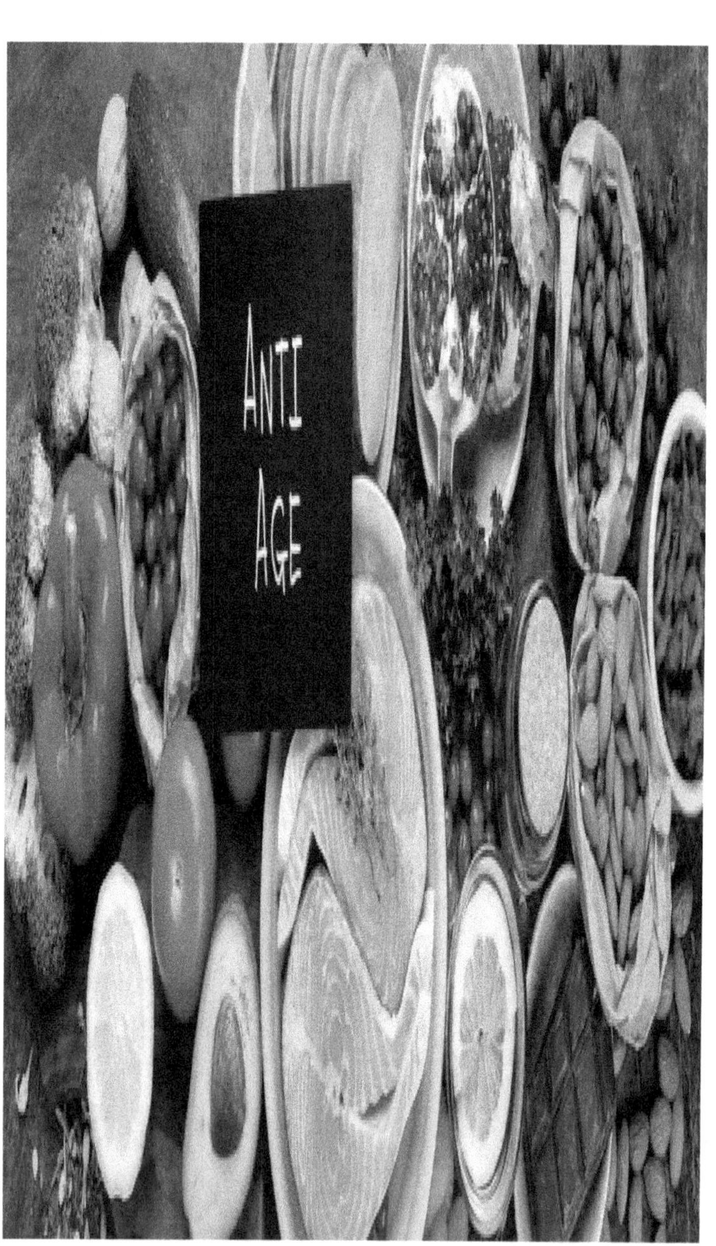

ANTI
AGE

CHAPTER 8

MAINTAINING A HEALTHY WEIGHT

Many women tend to ignore their weight. But do you know it is one of the most important factors in your long term health. Research has shown that weight is an important risk factor for many health problems like heart disease. Hypertension or high blood pressure, high cholesterol levels, diabetes, some cancers, joint problems or arthritis, gallstones, adolestent asthama, sleep asnea, and even snoring.

The weighing scale shows your weight but it does not measure your body fat or if you are at healthy weight. Your body is measured as a whole-all fat, muscle, organs, bone and water. Hence health professionals and personal trainer's advice against following just the weighing scale. According to experts, the body mass index (BMI), gives you a better idea if yoy are at a healthy weight and helps to determine whether or not you have a good body.

BMI is a calculation of your weight in relation to your height. It is calculated as (weight in kilograms)/height in meters2 and is interpreted as follows:

Below 18.5	Underweight
18.5 – 24.9	Normal
25 – 29.9	Overweight
30 and Above	Obese

Genetics also has an influence on weight but most of us can stay at a healthy weight by limiting what and how much we eat and doing regular physical activity like walking at a brisk pace, cycling, jogging or playing a sport such as tennis. Some experts think that the risk of diabetes, heart disease, and blood pressure begins to increase when the BMI goes above 22. So people with BMI less than 25 should avoid gaining weigjt and if possible work to lower the BMI to an optimal 22.

Besides BMI, the excess fat in abdomen also

increases your risk of cardiovascular disease, high blood pressure, and diabetes.

Age-related health problems in women can be avoided by maintaining a healthy weight. Women over 40 who are overweight or obese are at greater risk of developing a wide range of health problems, including diabetes, heart disease, stroke, and certain cancers. Additionally, being overweight can cause depression, fatigue, and other mental health issues.

To maintain a healthy weight, women over 40 should focus on eating a balanced diet full of whole grains, lean proteins, fruits, and vegetables. It can also be easier to maintain a healthy weight by eating smaller portions and avoiding processed foods, sugar, and saturated fat. Exercise is also an important part of staying healthy and maintaining a healthy weight. Attempt to engage in physical exercise most days of the week for at least 30 minutes.

It is also important to get regular health screenings and

to talk to your doctor about any changes in your body or health. Women over 40 should also get enough sleep and reduce stress levels to help maintain a healthy weight. Finally, women over 40 should remember to stay hydrated and drink plenty of water throughout the day. By maintaining a healthy weight and adopting a healthy lifestyle, women over 40 can reduce their risk of developing chronic health issues.

The following are exercise guidelines in maintaining a healthy weight:

1. **Include strength training:** Strength training is essential for all women, but especially for women over 40. Strength training helps build muscle, improve bone density, and boost metabolism. Aim for two to three days per week of strength training exercises using moderate to heavy weights.

2. **Incorporate cardio:** Cardio is important for overall heart health and for burning calories. It can assist in lowering the risk of diabetes, heart disease, and stroke.

Aim for at least 30 minutes of moderate-intensity cardio, such as walking, running, or swimming, at least five days per week.

3. **Stretch Regularly:** Stretching helps improve flexibility, reduce stress, and prevent injuries. Aim for at least 10 to 15 minutes of stretching each day, focusing on the muscles used in your strength training routine.

4. **Monitor Intensity:** As you age, your body may not be able to handle the same level of intensity as when you were younger. Monitor your intensity level and make sure you are not overdoing it.

5. **Stay Hydrated:** Proper hydration is essential for overall health, especially during exercise. It's crucial to drink water before, during, and after training.

Stress can also have an impact on weight, especially for women over 40. Stress can lead to overeating, which can lead to weight gain. Learning relaxation techniques and engaging in activities that reduce stress can help keep your weight in check. Getting adequate sleep is also important, as it can help reduce cravings for unhealthy foods. If you have added inches to your waistline over the years, its time you shed some inches by limiting your calorie intake and adding adequate exercise.

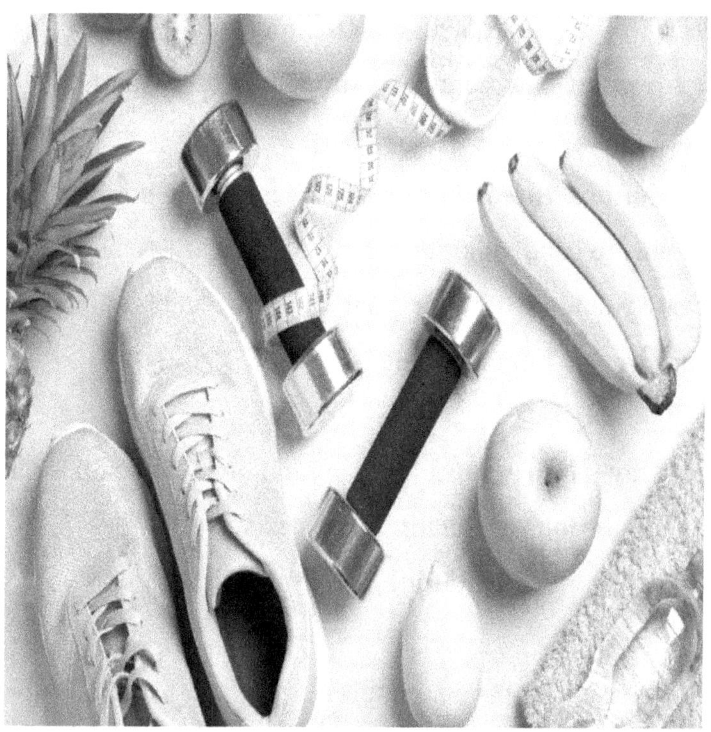

CHAPTER 9

MENTAL AND EMOTIONAL WELL-BEING

Mental and emotional well-being is the state of having a positive outlook on life and feeling good about yourself, your life, and your relationships with others. It is an important part of overall health and includes mental health, emotional health, and social health. Mental and emotional well-being means having a sense of purpose and meaning in life, feeling connected to others, and having a positive outlook. It is important to identify and address any mental health issues, as well as to make sure that your emotional needs are being met. Taking part in activities that make you happy, such as hobbies or spending time with friends and family, can help to maintain mental and emotional well-being.

Mental and emotional well-being are not the same as mental health, but they are closely related. Mental health includes the diagnosis and treatment of mental illnesses and disorders, while emotional well-being is about feeling good, having a positive outlook, and feeling connected to others. Mental and emotional well-being can be affected by a variety of factors, such as lifestyle, relationships, and environmental stressors. It is important to take steps to maintain mental and emotional well-being and to seek help if needed.

Mental and emotional well-being is an important factor in overall health, particularly for women over 40. As women age, they are more likely to experience depression and anxiety, as well as physical health issues. Mental and emotional health can be key factors in managing and preventing these physical health issues. Good mental and emotional health is about feeling good about oneself and having a positive outlook on life. It involves being emotionally resilient, being able to manage and cope with life's challenges, and having meaningful connections with others. It is important for women over 40 to take time for self-care, whether that is through relaxation, exercise, or other healthy activities.

When mental and emotional health is neglected, women over 40 may be at a higher risk of developing physical health problems, such as high blood pressure, heart disease, and diabetes. It is important to recognize the signs of depression, anxiety, and stress, and seek help if these issues persist. Talking to a therapist, doctor, or other health professional can help women over 40 manage these issues and reduce their risk of developing physical health problems.

Mental and emotional well-being can have a profound impact on the overall health of women over 40. It is important to take the time to focus on mental and emotional well-being in order to maintain physical health and lead a happy and fulfilling life.

By taking these necessary steps below to maintain mental and emotional well-being, women over 40 can decrease their risk of physical health problems and enjoy a better quality of life.

1. **Develop a consistent sleep schedule:** Make sure to get enough sleep each night and stick to a consistent bedtime and wake time.

2. **Eat healthy:** Eating a balanced and nutritious diet can help maintain mental and emotional well-being.

3. **Exercise regularly:** Regular physical activity can help to reduce stress, improve mood, and increase energy.

4. **Connect with others:** Make time for meaningful relationships with people who make you feel supported, valued, and appreciated.

5. **Practice self-care:** Take time to relax, practice mindfulness and meditation, and do activities that bring you joy.

6. **Seek professional help if needed:** If you are struggling with anxiety, depression, or other mental health issues, considers speaking to a therapist or mental health professional.

Therefore, mental and emotional well-being for women over 40 entails taking care of their physical, mental, and emotional health. This could include making sure to get adequate exercise, eating a healthy diet, getting enough sleep, managing stress, having meaningful relationships and social support, engaging in activities that bring joy, and finding time to relax and pursue hobbies. It also involves being mindful of your thoughts and emotions and seeking help when necessary. Additionally, engaging in activities that help you to build a positive self-image and self-esteem can help to promote mental and emotional wellbeing.

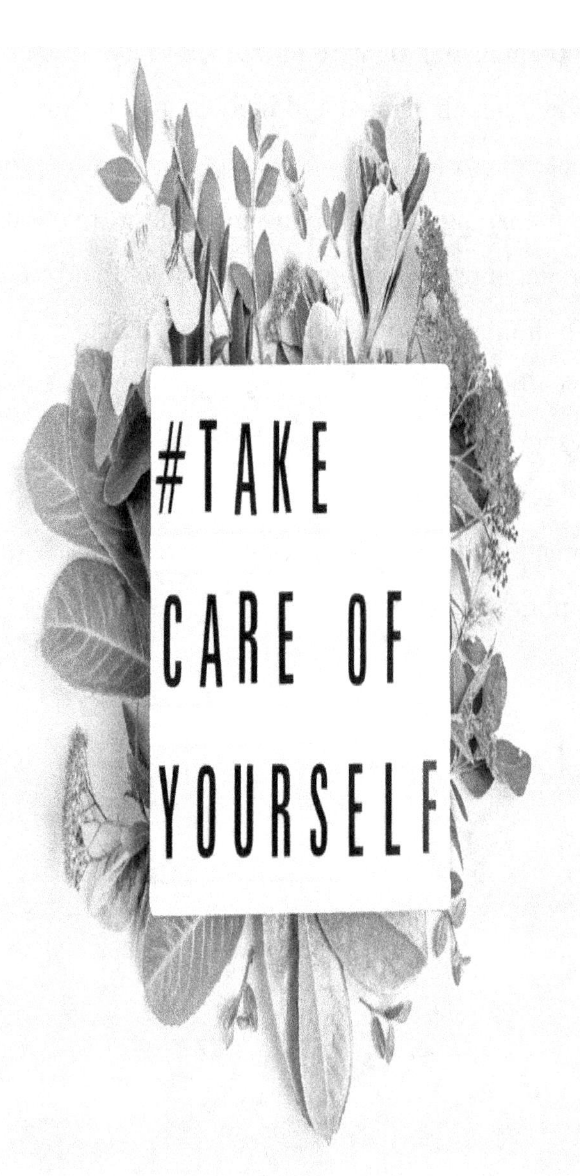
#TAKE
CARE OF
YOURSELF

CONCLUSION

Women over 40 have unique nutritional needs that must be addressed in order to stay healthy and vibrant. Eating a variety of nutrient-dense foods, limiting added sugar, and getting regular physical activity can help women over 40 meet their individual nutritional needs. Additionally, women over 40 should be aware of their risk of certain diet-related diseases, such as osteoporosis and heart disease, and take steps to prevent or manage these conditions. By following the guidelines stated in this book, women over 40 can maintain good health and a high quality of life for many years.

The journey to good nutrition for women over 40 can be both exciting and rewarding. With the right information, mindset, and resources enlisted in this book, women over 40 can embrace their unique nutritional needs and confidently take on the challenge of living a healthy life.

So, if you are a woman over 40, why not start your

journey to good nutrition today? With this little knowledge and support, you can make it happen and enjoy the many benefits of a healthier lifestyle.

Take the first step and make a commitment to yourself to strive for better health and nutrition. It's never too late to start living a healthier lifestyle, and you'll be amazed at how much better you can feel when you do.

So let's get started. It's time to make nutrition a priority and start living a healthier, more fulfilling life.